All About
STROKES

By Laura Flynn R.N., B.N., M.B.A., in consultation with her nurse educator associates and physicians who assisted in contributing and editing.

ISBN No: 978 1 896616 54 4

© 2016 Mediscript Communications Inc.

The publisher, Mediscript Communications Inc., acknowledges the financial support of the Government of Canada through the Canadian Book Fund for our publishing activities.

Printed in Canada

www.mediscript.net

Book and Front Cover design by:
Brian Adamson, www.AdamsonGraphics.net

S1002010

ALL ABOUT BOOKS

Trusted • Reliable • Certified

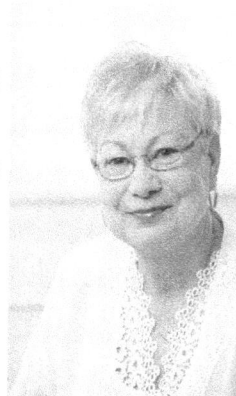

CONTENTS

INTRODUCTION

This book provides basic, non controversial and trusted information that can help a wide spectrum of readers.

The primary objective of the information is to help a person provide effective quality care to a loved one or someone in his or her care.

After reading this material you will have greater confidence in your caregiving role and will know what to do to help a person who suffered a stroke or is at risk of having one.

All the information is reliable and was written by a group of eminent nurse educators who ensured the information complies with best practice guidelines and satisfies the various accreditation and regulatory bodies. Because there is so much unreliable information on the internet, you can be assured the "All About" publications are HON (Health On the Net) certified.

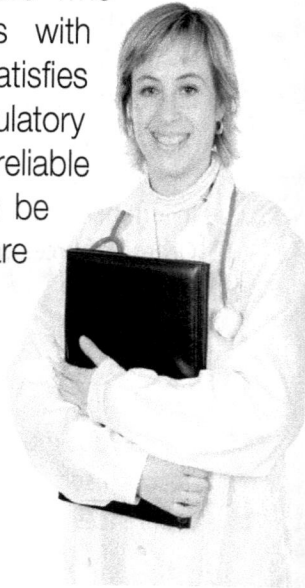

This book can be an invaluable aid to:

- A caregiver caring for a relative or friend;
- A health worker seeking a reference aid;
- Any person involved in health care wishing to expand his or her knowledge.

SOMETHING TO THINK ABOUT...

What we see depends mainly on
what we look for.

John Lubbock

AN IMPORTANT MESSAGE FROM THE PUBLISHER

Each person's treatment, advice, medical aids, physical therapy and other approaches to health care are unique and highly dependant upon the diagnosis and overall assessment by the medical team.

We emphasize therefore that the information within this book is not a substitute for the advice and treatment from a health care professional.

This book provides generic information concerning the issues around strokes and common sense, well-established care practices for people who have suffered strokes.

With all this in mind, the publishers and authors disclaim any responsibility for any adverse effects resulting directly or indirectly from the suggestions contained within this book or from any misunderstanding of the content on the part of the reader.

Three signs that mean you are getting older:

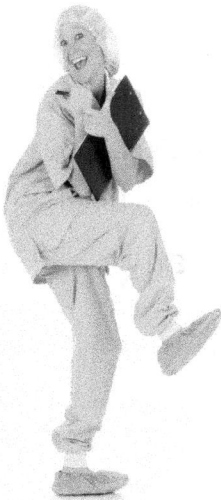

- Your back goes out more than you do.

- You enjoy hearing about other people's operations.

- You have a party and nobody calls the cops.

HOW MUCH DO YOU KNOW

It helps to figure out how much you know before starting. In this way you will have an idea as to the gaps in your knowledge prior to reading the content. Please circle to indicate the best answer. Remember, at this stage, you are not expected to know all the answers:

1. A stroke is usually the result of:

a. A clot in a blood vessel or artery of the brain

b. A clot in a blood vessel or artery of the heart

c. Bleeding in a blood vessel in the brain

d. A fall resulting in a head injury

2. Stroke is more common in:

a. High income earners

b. Older people

c. People who exercise often

d. People with a high level of education

3. A Transient Ischemic Attack (TIA) is considered to be:

a. A warning sign of a stroke

b. An interruption of blood to the heart

c. Permanently damaging

d. Another name for a stroke

4. Risk factors for a stroke include:

a. Blood type

b. Low blood cholesterol

c. Artery disease

d. Motor vehicle accidents

5. Symptoms of a stroke include:

a. Sudden severe headache

b. Prolonged weakness in both arms

c. A mild headache

d. Tiredness or fatigue

6. Which of the following is a controllable risk factor for stroke?

a. Heredity and race

b. High blood cholesterol

c. Gender

d. Previous stroke or heart attack

7. The effects of a stroke can include:

a. Arthritis

b. Depression

c. Increased energy level

d. Paralysis on both sides of the body

ANSWERS

1. a. A stroke is usually the result of a clot that forms in a blood vessel or artery in the brain. It can also occur when a blood vessel breaks and causes bleeding in the brain.

2. b. Although it can occur at any age, stroke is more common in people over 65 years.

3. a. A Transient Ischemic Attack (TIA) is a strong warning sign of a stroke. The more TIAs a person has, the greater the risk of a major stroke.

4. c. Narrowing of the carotid artery (the artery that supplies blood to the brain) increases the risk of stroke.

5. a. A sudden severe headache with no known cause is one of several symptoms of a possible stroke.

6. b. High blood cholesterol leads to the development of hardening of the arteries and increases the risk of stroke.

7. b. Most people experience a period of sadness following a stroke, which can develop into depression.

WHAT IS A STROKE?

Stroke (also called a "brain attack" or a "cerebrovascular accident") is the sudden interruption of blood flow to a part of the brain. Brain cells die due to a lack of oxygen and nutrients. Certain bodily functions (e.g. speech, balance, understanding, movement, and memory) that are controlled by the affected part of the brain can't work properly. The effects of a stroke depend upon where the brain was injured and how much damage occurred.

A stroke is usually the result of a clot that forms in a blood vessel or artery in the brain. It can also occur when a blood vessel breaks and causes bleeding in the brain. Stroke is more common in people over 65 years, although it can occur at any age. Injury from a stroke can be mild or severe and can have short-term or lasting effects.

DID YOU KNOW?

- Stroke is the 4th main cause of death in North America and the 3rd leading cause of death in the United States.

- About 700,000 Americans suffer from stroke each year.

- Stroke is the principal cause of long-term disability in North America.

WHAT IS A "TIA"?

A Transient Ischemic Attack (TIA) or "silent stroke" also involves an interruption of blood flow to the brain. A TIA, however, lasts for a shorter period of time; the symptoms begin suddenly but only last from a few minutes to a couple of hours and then disappear completely.

Although TIAs do not leave any permanent damage, they are a strong WARNING sign that a person may eventually have a stroke. The more TIAs a person has, the greater the risk of a major stroke.

The symptoms of a TIA are exactly the same as for a stroke. They can include muscle weakness down one side of the body, trouble speaking, vision problems, loss of balance, mood or personality changes and changes in sensation such as numbness.

WHAT ARE THE RISK FACTORS
FOR A STROKE?

Certain factors increase the risk of having a stroke. Some of these risk factors can be controlled, which means that you can do something to lower the risk. Others risk factors are uncontrollable; you can't do anything about uncontrollable risk factors.

UNCONTROLLABLE RISK FACTORS

AGE: The risk of stroke increases with age.

GENDER: Men are at increased risk of stroke. Women, however, live longer than men. With increasing age, the risk of dying from stroke increases. Women account for more than half of all the deaths from stroke.

HEREDITY AND RACE: The risk increases when there is a family history of stroke. Compared to Caucasians, African Americans are more likely to die from stroke. Stroke is the fourth main cause of death among Hispanics.

PREVIOUS STROKE OR HEART ATTACK: A previous stroke or a history of heart disease increases the risk of stroke.

ETHNICITY: Persons of certain ethnic groups (First Nations/Aboriginal Peoples and others of African, Hispanic, South Asian and Black descent) are at increased risk of getting high blood pressure and diabetes, conditions that can lead to stroke.

CONTROLLABLE RISK FACTORS

HIGH BLOOD PRESSURE: High blood pressure is the most important stroke risk factor that can be controlled. Many people with high blood pressure are not even aware that they have the condition. Everyone needs their blood pressure checked on a regular basis.

DIABETES: Persons with diabetes are at greater risk of stroke.

SMOKING: Smoking increases the risk of stroke quite a lot.

ARTERY DISEASE: Narrowing of the carotid artery (artery that supplies blood to the brain) increases the risk of stroke. Narrowing of the blood vessels that carry blood to the leg and arm muscles (peripheral artery disease) also increases the risk of stroke.

HEART DISEASE/ATRIAL FIBRILLATION: Atrial fibrillation is a disorder that affects the rhythm of the heart beat. It increases the likelihood that clots will form and cause a stroke. Heart disease also increases stroke risk.

TIA: A Transient Ischemic Attack is a warning sign of stroke.

CERTAIN BLOOD DISORDERS: Sickle cell disease, a genetic disease that mainly targets African Americans, increases the risk of stroke.

HIGH BLOOD CHOLESTEROL: High blood cholesterol leads to the development of a plaque along the walls of the blood vessels (also called "hardening of the arteries") and increases the risk of stroke.

INACTIVITY AND OBESITY: Lack of exercise and obesity increase the risk of stroke and of other conditions such as heart disease and diabetes.

HEAVY DRINKING: The increase in blood pressure that may result from heavy drinking raises the risk of stroke.

ILLEGAL DRUG USE: The use of certain illegal drugs, such as cocaine, has been linked to stroke and heart attacks.

Certain risk factors are unique to women. The use of oral contraceptives (birth control pills) increases the risk for certain women. Women who take birth control pills and who smoke, or those with other risk factors for stroke, are at greater risk for stroke. Pregnancy and childbirth increase the risk of stroke, although the overall risk is still low for women at this time of life. The risk of heart disease and stroke goes up after menopause.

CONSIDER FOR A MOMENT...

How many risk factors for stroke do you have?
What lifestyle changes can you make to decrease
your chances of having a stroke?

STROKE PREVENTION

Reducing even one risk factor can greatly decrease the chance of a stroke.

High blood pressure is the major controllable risk factor for stroke. Regular blood pressure checks are important since the condition often has no symptoms.

Regular medical checkups and a lifestyle that includes a healthy diet, regular exercise, and a healthy weight will also reduce the risk of stroke.

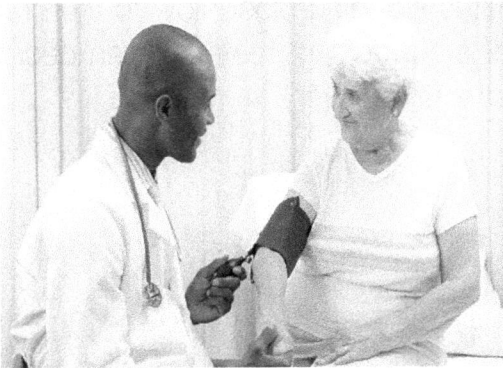

WHAT ARE THE SYMPTOMS OF A STROKE?

In 2003 the Canadian Stroke Network conducted a national survey to find out how much Canadians know about the disease. The results were shocking: 50% of those surveyed were unable to correctly describe what a stroke is. Almost half (48%) could not identify a single symptom of stroke. Reacting fast to signs of a stroke is very important. A stroke, like a heart attack, is a medical emergency. The person with signs of a stroke needs emergency medical assistance at once. Early treatment can often dissolve a clot that is stopping blood flow to the brain. Even a brief delay in getting treatment can decrease the chance of a full recovery.

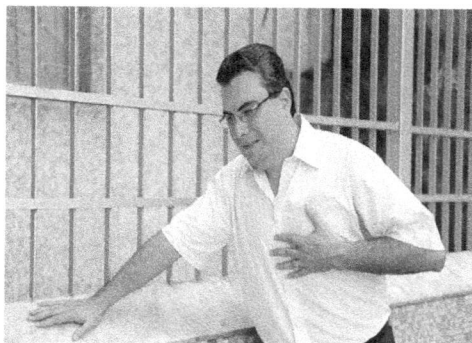

The warning signs of stroke are outlined below. A person could have several of these signs or just one:

- Sudden weakness or numbness in the face, arm or leg, particularly on one side of the body
- Sudden difficulty in speaking (i.e. talking or understanding)
- Sudden vision problems (i.e. loss of vision in one or both eyes, seeing double)
- Sudden loss of balance or coordination
- Sudden severe headache with no known cause

SOMETHING TO THINK ABOUT...

Some people think that a person is not seriously ill unless they have pain. Many persons who have a stroke, however, do not feel pain at the time.

LEFT SIDE BRAIN STROKE

When a stroke injures the left side of the brain, the right side of the body is affected. Symptoms such as weakness or paralysis on the right side of the body, difficulties with speech and language, and memory loss may occur. These clients may perform tasks slowly and carefully and have trouble with understanding.

RIGHT SIDE BRAIN STROKE

When a stroke affects the right side of the brain, the left side of the body is involved. Common symptoms are weakness or paralysis on the left side of the body, vision problems, and memory loss. Following a stroke on the right side of the brain, clients may be more impulsive in their actions. They may not be able to recognize the meaning of things that they see, smell, or hear and they may have difficulty with learning.

CONSIDER FOR A MOMENT...

Have you ever cared for someone following a stroke? If so, what symptoms did he or she have?

CARING FOR THE PERSON WITH A STROKE

Many people who've suffered strokes need help performing activities of daily living, such as eating, bathing, grooming, using the toilet and, in general, getting around.

Many different health professionals (such as a doctor, nurse, physiotherapist, occupational therapist, speech therapist, recreation therapist or social worker) may be involved in assisting the person to recovery. The person's family also plays an important part in the process. Recovery involves having the person:

- Maintain abilities that are present

- Relearn skills that have been lost

- Make up for losses that may be temporary or permanent

The goal in recovery is to encourage people to do their best in all aspects of life.

HOW TO HELP

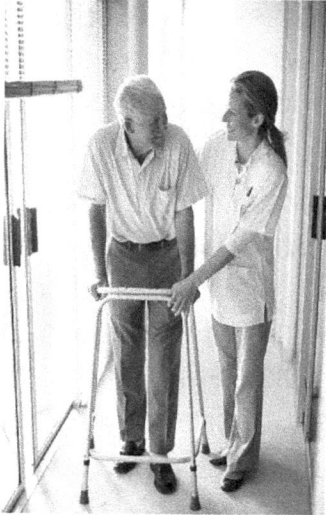

You can assist with activities of daily living while helping the person in your care to become as independent as possible. In many cases, becoming more independent will mean learning how to do things differently.

For example, walking may still be possible but only with the use of a cane or a walker. Dressing may require the use of special Velcro fasteners for clothing, elastic pants, and slip-on shoes. Weighted utensils may help the person to eat independently. A raised toilet seat and safety rail may make toileting alone possible.

If you are caring for someone in her home, changes may have to be made to the home environment. These changes include use of non-slip mats, extra railing in the hallways, grab bars, and widening of the bathroom door.

Family members who are heavily involved in caring for their loved ones should take a break from continuing care. It's important that caregivers take care of their own physical and emotional health.

Groups that provide support and information for people recovering from stroke and their families are present in many local areas. The section "Other Resources" outlines some of these information sources. The local health authority may also be able to provide information about support group meetings.

CONSIDER FOR A MOMENT...

Which support groups for stroke

victims and their families are

present in your area?

POSITIONING AND SKIN CARE

Skin care and proper positioning are very important following a stroke. Without it, the person in your care may be prone to pressure sores and contractures (shortening and tightening of muscles).

You may have to assist with turning and positioning every couple of hours. Injuries to the side affected by the stroke are quite common during transfer and positioning.

You must be very careful when moving the person. Use pillows, rolled blankets, and other devices to support and position the affected side properly while he or she is in bed or in a chair.

Special pressure-reducing mattresses can make the person more comfortable and help prevent skin breakdown.

EMOTIONS

Following a stroke, a person may be very emotional and react in ways that do not 'fit' with the situation. He or she may laugh or cry at odd times and act differently than before the stroke occurred. Someone who avoided foul language in the past may now swear often.

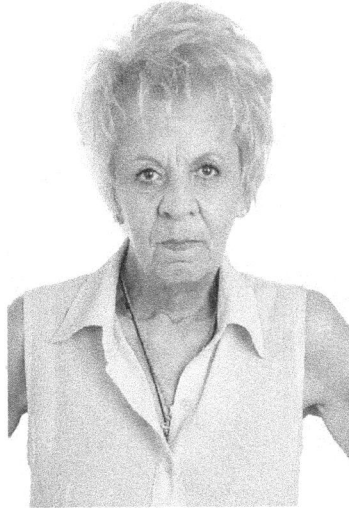

These reactions can be very hard on the family. They need to be reminded that the behaviors are a result of the injury and are not within the person's control. Ignore behaviors that are not appropriate and advise the family to do so as well. As time goes on, your client may have greater command of emotions.

Frustration is a very common emotion following a stroke. Learning how to eat, dress, walk, and toilet again can be very slow and difficult. Offer support and encouragement. If you notice that the person is tired or frustrated while trying to learn a task, suggest taking a break. You can try again later when he or she is rested.

Most people go through a period of sadness as they come to terms with all the losses they have had because of a stroke. Sometimes the sadness develops into a depression that interferes with health and progress. Referral to a psychologist, social worker, or doctor may be necessary. Medication may be needed to offset feelings of depression.

APHASIA
(COMMUNICATING PROBLEMS)

Not being able to communicate well is probably one of the most frustrating challenges that a person can face; yet it is a common problem following a stroke. Aphasia is a type of communication problem that affects the ability to speak, read, write, or understand what others are saying.

The impact of aphasia can be mild or severe. Some people recover quickly from aphasia. Others have ongoing problems.

In one type of aphasia (expressive aphasia), the person can understand others but cannot express himself/herself well. Reading may not be a problem, although writing is sometimes affected. The person's words do not coincide with his/her thoughts. For example, he may want a glass of water but ask for a book instead. Speech may be jumbled and slurred. The person with expressive aphasia is often aware of the mistakes he is making.

The person with receptive aphasia will have difficulty with understanding language but may speak without effort. Many of the words spoken will not be correct. It is not uncommon for people to have problems with both speaking and understanding (expressive-receptive aphasia).

Communication problems resulting from aphasia can be very different. What works for one person may not work for another. A team of professionals may work together to develop a communication plan for a particular person. Follow the care plan to find out how you should communicate with the person in your care.

Having aphasia does not mean that the person is "feeble-minded". Don't ignore your aphasic patient. Treat the person with the same respect you would show to any other adult.

Here are several methods that have been found helpful in general when communicating with a person with aphasia:

- Speak clearly and slowly.

- Keep your sentences short and simple.

- Take your time. If the person feels that you are hurried, he/she may not even want to try to communicate with you.

- Be supportive and encouraging. A relaxed setting works best.

- Remind the person in your care and her family that improvement in communication can sometimes continue for quite some time after the stroke has taken place.

- Encourage the person to speak to you. Consider stopping if he becomes very frustrated or tired.

- Use gestures and pointing while talking.

- Give the person lots of time to understand what you have said and to answer. Although it is generally better not to respond for the person, there may be times when it will be less frustrating for him or her if you do so.

- Give one direction at a time.

- Name the objects you are using while assisting with bathing, grooming, and other activities of daily living.

- Repeat what you have said to ensure understanding.

- Try using a picture board or printed materials.

- Encourage the person to get lots of rest. People who have had a stroke usually tire easily which makes communication more difficult.

KEEP IN MIND...

Communication involves more than the use of words. We also communicate through the tone and pitch of our voices, body posture, eye movements, and facial expression. How you express yourself without words is just as important as what you say.

Observe the other person, as well, for these nonverbal cues. Communication can be more effective if the person in your care feels that you have a sense of what he/she is going through and that you genuinely care.

A common mistake when caring for aphasic patients is to think that they understand more than they actually do. It's always a good idea to check how well the person understands you. Keep in mind that people often get stuck on a word or idea in the recovery phase, so it is important to keep questions and directions simple and clear.

Sometimes a person may get confused over yes and no answers. Carefully watch for facial expressions and other body language to get a better understanding of the person's needs.

CONSIDER FOR A MOMENT...

Have you ever cared for someone with aphasia?

If so, what worked well during your communications with him or her?

What didn't work as well, and

why do you think that was?

DYSPHAGIA (SWALLOWING PROBLEMS)

Difficulty swallowing, or dysphagia, affects 30-60% of people who have had a stroke. Dysphagia can cause fluid or food to enter the airway, resulting in serious problems such as choking and pneumonia.

Observe the person in your care for signs that dysphagia may be present. Some common signs are coughing while eating or drinking, pocketing of food (food in the mouth after swallowing), breathing difficulties while eating, taking a long time to chew food, and frequent clearing of the throat. If signs of dysphagia are present, the doctor should be notified.

Here are several techniques that can be helpful when feeding the person with dysphagia:

- Position him in an upright sitting position for meals.

- Encourage self-feeding, if possible, so that she has more control while eating.

- Avoid the use of straws so that he has more control while drinking.

- Avoid bland foods.

- Give a soft diet.

- Place foods in the unaffected side of the mouth.

- Give small bites and encourage the person to chew well.

- Offer liquids following, not during, the meal.

- Do not serve food or liquids (especially water) at a lukewarm temperature.

- Encourage the person to sweep the mouth with a finger after eating if food pocketing occurs.

- Keep her sitting for 30-45 minutes after the meal.

Different kinds of swallowing problems exist so that soft foods may not always be recommended. Likewise, sitting up while eating may not work best in every situation. A speech therapist, dietitian, occupational therapist, nurse, or other health care professional can assess to develop a specific plan to help with the problem.

INCONTINENCE

Urinary incontinence is the involuntary loss of urine that is sufficient to be considered a problem. It often results in a person being placed into a nursing home. Urinary incontinence is a common condition following a stroke, however, and can often improve with proper treatment.

The treatment plan for the person in your care will depend on the results of an assessment and evaluation of the condition. Sometimes a urologist (a doctor who specializes in problems involving the urinary tract) does this assessment. Other professionals, such as a nurse, occupational therapist, or physiotherapist may be involved. Surgery, special exercises, or medications are used for some types of incontinence. An indwelling catheter is also used at times but should not be a first choice due to the risk of infection with short and long-term use. Follow the instructions of the continence specialist with respect to treatment of the condition.

Bladder training is used for some persons following a stroke. Bladder training involves slowly increasing or shortening the time between toileting. It may involve keeping a record of the times that the person voids (urinates) for several days and then planning toileting around that time. If a record cannot be developed, you may be asked to assist the person to void every one to two hours at specific times and then encourage him/her to slowly increase the length of time between each voiding.

Encourage complete emptying of the bladder each time the person goes to the bathroom. Certain substances, such as tea, coffee, chocolate, alcohol, or spicy foods increase the urge to void and may have to be eliminated or used in moderation. To avoid problems at night, cut down on the amount of fluids given in the evening.

OTHER RESOURCES

The following associations can provide information about stroke to patients, families and professionals:

American Heart Association
National Center
7272 Greenville Avenue
Dallas, TX 75231
AHA: 1-800-AHA-USA-1
or 1-800-242-8721
http://www.americanheart.org/
A national voluntary health agency whose mission is to reduce disability and death from cardiovascular diseases and stroke.

American Stroke Association
National Center
7272 Greenville Avenue
Dallas TX 75231
ASA: 1-888-4-STROKE
or 1-888-478-7653
http://www.strokeassociation.org/
Maintains a listing of support groups for stroke survivors, their families, friends and interested professionals. Publishes Stroke Connection magazine, a forum for stroke survivors and their families to share information about coping with strokes.

Heart and Stroke Foundation of Canada
222 Queen St., Ste 1402
Ottawa ON K1P 5V9
Tel: 613-569-4361
Fax: 613-569-3278
http://ww2.heartandstroke.ca/
A national voluntary non-profit organization that aims to improve the health of Canadians by preventing and reducing disability and death from heart disease and stroke. Involved in research, health promotion and advocacy.

National Stroke Association
9707 E. Easter Lane
Englewood, Co. 80112
Toll Free: 1-800-STROKES
Phone: 303-649-9299
http://www.stroke.org
Aims to reduce the incidence and impact of stroke through prevention, medical treatment, rehabilitation, family support and research.

CASE EXAMPLE

Dorothy Brown, an 84-year old woman you are caring for of yours, recently had a stroke that left her with paralysis on the right side of her body and severe aphasia. One side of her face now droops and she drools constantly. You are present on the day that, Anna, Mrs. Brown's sister, visits for the first time following the stroke. After several attempts to have a conversation with her sister fail, Anna suddenly jumps up and leaves the room in a hurry. You notice that she is crying.

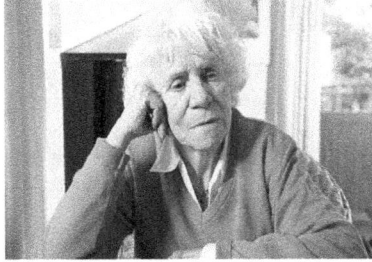

What could you say to Anna to help in this situation?

YOUR ANSWERS TO CASE EXAMPLE

SUGGESTED ANSWERS TO CASE EXAMPLE

Anna is obviously quite upset. This is the first time that she has seen her sister since the stroke. She is probably feeling shocked and frightened by the change in her sister's manner and appearance.

You can help Anna on her next visit by letting her voice her concerns. You might suggest that Anna visit for short periods of time at first until she feels more comfortable being around her sister again.

The ability to communicate following a stroke can improve over time for many people. As well, depending on the type of aphasia that Mrs. Brown has, she may be able to understand the spoken word even though she can't communicate well. Her doctor (or communication team members) may be able to give Anna more information about that aspect of her sister's care. They may also be able to give her helpful tips that can help with communication.

Anna may also benefit from learning more about stroke. Tell her where she can go to get information about it (see "Other Resources"). Many people find it helpful to join a support group. Tell Anna about support groups offered in your area for families of stroke victims.

CONCLUSION

Caring for a person who has had a stroke presents many challenges for caregivers. You can help in this difficult situation by offering support and reassurance to the person and his or her family. Both you and family members need frequent breaks to ensure that you can be physically and emotionally healthy to care for your client or loved one. Various support groups offer help for clients, families and caregivers.

Be patient and understanding while encouraging people to regain and improve functions that were lost due to stroke. Report any changes in the person's condition immediately. Working toward healthy goals to succeed in the activities of daily living should start immediately after a stroke.

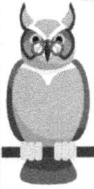

CHECK YOUR KNOWLEDGE

1. Explain the meaning of the word "stroke".

2. Name the risk factors for a stroke.

3. Identify the warning signs of a stroke.

4. List five possible problems that can result from a stroke.

5. Give four techniques that may be helpful when communicating with an aphasic person.

6. List three techniques that may be helpful when feeding the person with dysphagia.

TEST YOURSELF

Please circle to indicate the best answer:

1. Stroke is:

a. Also known as a "Cardiovascular Accident"

b. The main cause of death in Canada

c. A condition that can affect people of all ages

d. A principal cause of short-term disability in North America

2. Aphasia is a problem involving:

a. Language

b. Walking

c. Feeding

d. Thinking

3. Which are common symptoms when a stroke affects the left side of the brain?

a. Impulsive behaviour

b. Vision problems

c. Weakness or paralysis on the right side of the body

d. Weakness or paralysis on the left side of the body

4. Difficulty swallowing is also known as:

a. Dysphagia

b. Aphasia

c. Brain attack

d. Receptive aphasia

5. Which strategy is helpful when caring for a client with dysphagia?

a. Offer bland foods

b. Encourage self-feeding

c. Place food in the affected side of mouth

d. Offer liquids during a meal when feeding

6. Bladder training, following a stroke, involves:

a. Voiding at specific times during the day

b. Increasing fluid intake at bedtime

c. Holding urine for as long as possible

d. Drinking certain substances such as coffee and alcohol

7. The following may help when communicating with an aphasic person:

a. Speak in a loud tone of voice

b. Use gestures as you speak

c. Give several directions at a time

d. Make the person feel hurried to motivate them

ANSWERS

1. c. Although stroke is more common in people over 65 years, it can occur at any age.

2. a. Aphasia is a type of communication problem that affects the ability to speak, read, write, or understand what others are saying.

3. c. When a stroke injures the left side of the brain, the right side of the body is affected.

4. a. Dysphagia can cause fluid or food to enter the airway, resulting in serious problems such as choking and pneumonia.

5. b. Self-feeding will allow the dysphagic person to have more control while eating.

6. a. Bladder training involves slowly increasing or shortening the time between toileting. It may involve keeping a record of the times that the person voids for several days and then planning toileting around that time.

7. b. Using gestures and pointing has been found to be helpful when communicating with the aphasic person.

REFERENCES

American Heart Association (2005). Stroke risk factors. Retrieved August 6, 2005 from http://www.americanheart.org/presenter.jhtml?identifier=4716

American Stroke Association (2005a). Impact of stroke. Retrieved August 6, 2005 from http://www.strokeassociation.org/presenter.jhtml?identifier=1033

American Stroke Association (2005b). Stroke among Hispanics. Retrieved August 8, 2005 from http://www.strokeassociation.org/presenter.jhtml?identifier=3030389

American Stroke Association (2005c). Learn to recognize a stroke. Retrieved August 8, 2005 from http://www.strokeassociation.org/presenter.jhtml?identifier=1020

American Stroke Association (2005d). What are the effects of stroke? Retrieved August 8, 2005 from http://www.strokeassociation.org/presenter.jhtml?identifier=1052

Canadian Stroke Network (2005). Retrieved August 7, 2005 from http://www.canadianstrokenetwork.ca/aboutus/success/survey.php

Galvan, T. J. (2001). Dysphagia: going down and staying down. American Journal of Nursing, 101 (1), 37-43.

Heart and Stroke Foundation of Canada. (2003). Stroke risk factors. Retrieved August 6, 2005 from http://ww2. heartandstroke.ca/Page.asp?PageID=33&ArticleID=438&Src= stroke&From=SubCategory

Heart and Stroke Foundation of Canada. (2002). Stroke statistics. Retrieved August 6, 2005 from http://ww2. heartandstroke.ca/Page.asp?PageID=1613&ContentID=1934 7&ContentTypeID=1

Ignatavicius, D. & Workman, M. (Eds.), (2002). Medical-surgical nursing: Critical thinking for collaborative care. Philadelphia: Saunders.

Mower, D. M. (1997). Brain attack. Nursing, 27 (3), 34-39.

Rice, R. (2000). Manual of home health nursing procedures (2nd ed.). St. Louis, MO: Mosby.

Sorrentino, S. (2004). Mosby's Canadian textbook for the support worker. Toronto, ON: Mosby.

Sundin, K., Jansson, L., & Norberg, A. (2000). Communicating with people with stroke and aphasia: understanding through sensation without words. Journal of Clinical Nursing, 9, 481-488.

Travers, P. L. (1999). Poststroke dysphagia: implications for nurses. Rehabilitation Nursing, 24 (2), 69-73.